MW00737218

Every Decker book is accompanied by a CD-ROM.

BC Decker pioneered the concept of providing high-quality electronic publications to accompany the traditional text format of presenting clinical information to readers. The commitment to innovation and excellence continues.

Treatment of Common Oral Conditions includes a dual-platform CD-ROM featuring bonus multiple-choice questions designed to reinforce the treatment modalities outlined in the text. The fully searchable PDF files of the complete text and downloadable images facilitate the exploration of need-to-know information and are an ideal medium for patient education.

The book and disc are sold only as a package; neither is available independently. We trust you will find the book/CD package an invaluable resource; your comments and suggestions are most welcome.

Please visit www.bcdecker.com for a complete list of titles in your discipline. Our innovative approach to providing powerful informational tools for healthcare professionals means that Decker products belong in your library, and on your hard drive.

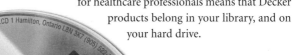

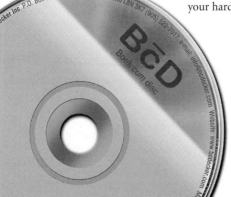

Brian C. Decker
CEO and Publisher

CLINICIAN'S GUIDES

The *Clinician's Guide* Series is another AAOM educational service. The other Clinician's Guides available from the Academy include:

Treatment of Common Oral Conditions, 6/e
Tobacco Cessation
Oral Health in Geriatric Patients, 2/e
Pharmacology
Chronic Orofacial Pain, 2/e
Oral Cancer
Oral Diseases in Children

CLINICIAN'S GUIDE

Treatment of

Common Oral Conditions

Sixth Edition

Michael A. Siegel, DDS, MS
Professor and Chair
Department of Diagnostic Sciences
Nova Southeastern University College of Dental Medicine
Fort Lauderdale, Florida

Sol Silverman Jr, MA, DDS
Professor
Division of Oral Medicine
Department of Orofacial Sciences
University of California School of Dentistry
San Francisco, California

Thomas P. Sollecito, DMD
Associate Dean for Academic Affairs
Associate Professor of Oral Medicine
Department of Oral Medicine
University of Pennsylvania School of Dental Medicine
Philadelphia, Pennsylvania

2006
BC Decker Inc
Hamilton

BC Decker Inc.
P.O. Box 620, L.C.D. 1
Hamilton, Ontario L8N 3K7
Tel: 905-522-7017; 800-568-7281
Fax: 905-522-7839; 888-311-4987
email: info@bcdecker.com
Website: www.bcdecker.com

© 2006 BC Decker Inc.
All rights reserved

All rights reserved. No part of this publication may be reproduced, stored in a retrieval system,
or transmitted, in any form or by any means, electronic, mechanical, photocopying, recording,
or otherwise, without prior written permission from the publisher.

08 09 10 11 12 / WPC /10 9 8 7 6 5 4 3 2
ISBN 978-1-55009-323-0
Printed in the United States by Walsworth Printing Company

Sales and Distribution

United States
BC Decker Inc
P.O. Box 785
Lewiston, NY 14092-0785
Tel: 905-522-7017; 800-568-7281
Fax: 905-522-7839; 888-311-4987
E-mail: info@bcdecker.com
www.bcdecker.com

Canada
McGraw-Hill Ryerson Education
Customer Care
300 Water St.
Whitby, Ontario   L1N 9B6
Tel: 1-800-565-5758
Fax: 1-800-463-5885

Foreign Rights
John Scott & Company
International Publishers' Agency
P.O. Box 878
Kimberton, PA 19442
Tel: 610-827-1640
Fax: 610-827-1671
E-mail: jsco@voicenet.com

Japan
United Publishers Services Limited
1-32-5 Higashi-Shinagawa
Shinagawa-Ku, Tokyo 140-0002
Tel: 03 5479 7251
Fax: 03 5479 7307

UK, Europe, Middle East
McGraw-Hill Education
Shoppenhangers Road
Maidenhead
Berkshire, England SL6 2QL
Tel: 44-0-1628-502500
Fax: 44-0-1628-635895
www.mcgraw-hill.co.uk

Singapore, Malaysia, Thailand, Philippines, Indonesia, Vietnam, Pacific Rim, Korea
McGraw-Hill Education
60 Tuas Basin Link
Singapore 638775
Tel: 65-6863-1580
Fax: 65-6862-3354

Australia, New Zealand
McGraw-Hill Australia
Pty LtdLevel 2, 82 Waterloo RoadNorth Ryde, NSW,
2113Australia
Customer Service AustraliaPhone: +61 (2) 9900 1800
Fax: +61 (2) 9900 1980
Email: cservice_sydney@mcgraw-hill.com

Customer Service New Zealand
Phone (Free Phone): +64 (0) 800 449 312
Fax (Free Phone): +64 (0) 800 449 318
Email: cservice@mcgraw-hill.co.nz

Brazil
Tecmedd Importadora E Distribuidora De Livros Ltda.
Avenida Maurílio Biagi, 2850
City Ribeirão, Ribeirão Preto – SP – Brasil
CEP: 14021-000
Tel: 0800 992236
Fax: (16) 3993-9000
E-mail: tecmedd@tecmedd.com.br

India, Bangladesh, Pakistan, Sri Lanka
CBS Publishers & Distributors
4596/1A-11, Darya Ganj
New Delhi-2, India
Tel: 23271632
Fax: 23276712
E-mail: cbspubs@vsnl.com

Notice: The authors and publisher have made every effort to ensure that the patient care recommended herein, including choice of drugs and drug dosages, is in accord with the accepted standard and practice at the time of publication. However, since research and regulation constantly change clinical standards, the reader is urged to check the product information sheet included in the package of each drug, which includes recommended doses, warnings, and contraindications. This is particularly important with new or infrequently used drugs. Any treatment regimen, particularly one involving medication, involves inherent risk that must be weighed on a case-by-case basis against the benefits anticipated. The reader is cautioned that the purpose of this book is to inform and enlighten; the information contained herein is not intended as, and should not be employed as, a substitute for individual diagnosis and treatment.

DEDICATION

The Editors wish to dedicate this volume to our wives Sharon, Betty, and Carolyn to recognize their unconditional love, friendship, inspiration, and support.

This sixth edition is also dedicated to the memory of William K. Bottomley, DDS, MS, whose educational foresight served as the original inspiration for this monograph and who served as an original coeditor of the first three editions of this monograph, for his contributions to the American Academy of Oral Medicine and to oral medicine education.

CONTENTS

CONTRIBUTING AUTHORS

Contributing authors are members of the American Academy of Oral Medicine. This monograph represents a consensus of the contributing authors and not necessarily the private views of any of the individuals.

Robert N. Arm, DMD

Ronald Brown, DDS, MS

Joseph D'Ambrosio, DDS, MS

Joel B. Epstein, DMD, MS

Catherine M. Flaitz, DDS, MS

Michael Glick, DMD

Martin S. Greenberg, DDS

Miriam Grushka, DDS, PhD

Jed J. Jacobson, DDS, MPH

Joseph L. Konzelman, DDS

Francina Lozada-Nur, DDS, MS, MPH

Cesar A. Migliorati, DDS, MS, PhD

Craig S. Miller, DMD, MS

Abdel R. Mohammad, DDS, MS, MPH

Brian C. Muzyka, DMD

Douglas E. Peterson, DMD, PhD

Abraham Reiner, DDS

Nelson L. Rhodus, DMD, MPH

Jonathan A. Ship, DMD

Martin T. Tyler, DDS, MEd

AMERICAN ACADEMY OF ORAL MEDICINE

Oral medicine is the specialty of dentistry responsible for the oral health care of medically compromised patients and for the diagnosis and management of medically related disorders or conditions affecting the oral and maxillofacial region.

GOAL: Oral medicine seeks to improve the quality of life of ambulatory and nonambulatory patients with chronic, recurrent, and medically related disorders of the oral and maxillofacial region.

SCOPE: Oral medicine is a nonsurgical specialty that includes the physical evaluation, diagnosis, and therapeutic management of and research into medically related oral diseases such as

1. Oral mucosal, salivary gland and functional disorders of the stomatognathic system
2. Chemosensory and neurologic impairment of the oral and maxillofacial complex
3. Orofacial disorders and complications resulting from systemic disease, aging, immunosuppression, and, secondary to drug side effects, radiotherapy, chemotherapy, and hospitalization

AAOM ORAL MEDICINE VISION STATEMENT

The practice of oral medicine enables optimal health to all people through the diagnosis and management of oral diseases. Fundamental to this vision are

- Recognition of the interaction of oral and systemic health
- Integration of medicine and oral health care
- Management of pharmacotherapeutics necessary for treatment of oral and systemic diseases
- Investigation of the etiology and treatment of oral diseases through basic science, oral epidemiology, and clinical research
- Research, teaching, and patient care
- Provision of care for medically complex patients, the elderly, and those undergoing cancer therapy
- Prevention, diagnosis, and management for the following disorders to include salivary gland diseases, orofacial pain and other neurosensory disorders, and oral mucous membranes

The American Academy of Oral Medicine (AAOM) achieves these goals by holding one or more national meetings annually; by presenting lectures, workshops, and seminars; by promoting research excellence by sponsoring the Lester Burket Student Award and the Robert I. Schattner Abstract Presentations; by sponsoring a section in the *Journal of Oral Surgery, Oral Medicine, Oral Pathology, Oral Radiology and Endodontics*; and by sponsorships of the American Board of Oral Medicine and the Oral Medicine Research Foundation, Inc.

Acknowledgments

The American Academy of Oral Medicine wishes to thank Drs. Michael Glick, Jeff Casiglia, and Francina Lozada-Nur for their hours of review and revision.

INTRODUCTION

This monograph is intended as a quick reference to the etiologic factors, clinical description, currently accepted therapeutic management, and patient education of the more common oral conditions.

All recommended treatments were current at the time of the publication of this guide. However, new medications are constantly made available to the clinician and therapeutic strategies evolve as new knowledge becomes known. The prudent clinician is well advised to consider this when using this guide.

Some of the recommended treatments have been more thoroughly investigated than others, but all have been reported to be of clinical value.

For many conditions described in this monograph, there is currently no cure, but there are treatment modalities that can relieve discomfort, shorten the clinical duration and frequency, and minimize recurrences.

Clinicians are reminded that an accurate diagnosis is imperative for clinical success.

Every effort should be made to determine the diagnosis prior to initiating treatment. Infection and malignancy must be ruled out. Where signs, symptoms, and microscopic and other laboratory evidence do not support a definitive diagnosis, empirical treatment may be initiated and evaluated as a therapeutic trial. Further treatment can be determined by the patient's response. However, when healing of a lesion or when an expected response to treatment is not achieved within an expected period of time, a biopsy is recommended.

Patient management should be governed by the natural history of the oral condition and the fact that there is either a palliative, supportive, or curative treatment.

Referral of patients should be made when the patient's problems are beyond the scope of the clinician.

All drugs require a prescription unless identified as over-the-counter (OTC) drugs. Please note that the Food and Drug Administration (FDA) has been active in recent years with allowing OTC status for drugs formerly available by prescription only. Be sure to check on the dosages of the newly released (OTC) drugs because they are usually of a different strength than those available by prescription.

The literature accompanying the prescription topical medications suggested in this guide may recommend "for external use only." The oral cavity is completely lined with keratinized or nonkeratinized squamous epithelium that is classified as ectoderm, an external body covering. It is therefore acceptable to use topical medications intraorally as recommended in this guide.

We hope you will find this monograph a useful resource in your daily practice.

For the Editors,
Michael A. Siegel
Fort Lauderdale 2006

STANDARD ABBREVIATIONS

i	one
ii	two
iii	three
ā	before
ac	before meals (ante cibum)
ad lib	as desired (ad libitum)
asap	as soon as possible
AAOM	American Academy of Oral Medicine
bid	twice a day (bis in die)
btl	bottle
c̄	with
cap	capsule
CBC	complete blood count
CDC	United States Centers for Disease Control and Prevention
crm	cream
disp	dispense on a prescription label
elix	elixir
FDA	United States Food and Drug Administration
g	gram
gtt	drop
h	hour
hs	at bedtime (hora somni)
HSV	herpes simplex virus
IU	international unit
IV	intravenous
L	liter
liq	liquid
loz	lozenge
mg	milligram
min	minute
mL	milliliter
NaF	sodium fluoride
oint	ointment
OTC	over-the-counter
oz	ounce
p	after
pc	after meals (post cibum)

PABA	para-aminobenzoic acid
PHN	postherpetic neuralgia
PLT	platelet count
po	by mouth (per os)
prn	as needed (pro re nata)
q	every
q2h	every 2 hours
q4h	every 4 hours
q6h	every 6 hours
q8h	every 8 hours
q12h	every 12 hours
qam	every morning
qd	every day (quaque die)
qhs	every bedtime
qid	four times a day (quarter in die)
qod	every other day
qpm	every evening
qsad	add a sufficient quantity to equal
qwk	every week
RAS	recurrent aphthous stomatitis
RAU	recurrent aphthous ulcer
RBC	red blood cell count
RHL	recurrent herpes labialis
RIH	recurrent intraoral herpes
Rx	prescription
ś	without
Sig	patient dosing instructions on prescription label
sol	solution
SPF	sun protection factor
stat	immediately
syr	syrup
tab	tablet
tbsp	tablespoon
tid	three times a day (ter in die)
top	topical
tsp	teaspoon
U	unit
ut dict	as directed (ut dictum)
UV	ultraviolet
visc	viscous
VZV	varicella-zoster virus
WBC	white blood cell count
wk	week
yr	year
Zn	zinc

BURNING MOUTH DISORDER

ETIOLOGY

Multiple conditions have been implicated in the causation of burning mouth disorder. Current literature favors neurogenic, vascular, and psychogenic etiologies. However, other conditions, such as xerostomia, candidosis, referred pain from the tongue musculature, chronic infections, reflux of gastric acid, medications, blood dyscrasias, nutritional deficiencies, hormonal imbalances, and allergic and inflammatory disorders, need to be considered.

CLINICAL DESCRIPTION

Burning mouth disorder is characterized by the absence of clinical signs (Figure 1-1).

RATIONALE FOR TREATMENT

To reduce discomfort by addressing possible etiologic factors.

TREATMENT

It is of the utmost importance to reassure the patient that this disorder is not infectious or contagious and does not progress to a premalignant or malignant condition.

On the basis of history, physical evaluation, and specific laboratory studies, rule out all possible organic etiologies. Minimal blood studies should include CBC

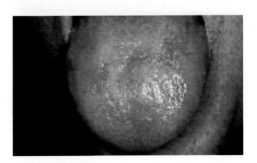

FIGURE 1-1

Normal appearance of the tongue in a female patient complaining of chronic lingual burning. Her symptoms were controlled with chlordiazepoxide (Librium).

and differential, fasting glucose, iron, ferritin, folic acid and vitamin B$_{12}$, and a thyroid profile (thyroid-stimulating hormone, triiodothyronine, thyroxine).

> **Rx:** Diphenhydramine (Children's Benadryl) elix 12.5 mg/5 mL (OTC).
> Disp: 1 btl.
> Sig: Rinse with 1 tsp (5 mL) for 2 minutes before each meal and swallow. Children's Benadryl is alcohol free.

When the burning mouth is considered psychogenic or idiopathic, tricyclic antidepressants or benzodiazepines in low doses exhibit the properties of analgesia and sedation and are frequently successful in reducing or eliminating the symptoms after several weeks or months. The dosage is adjusted according to patient reaction and clinical symptomatology. The following five systemic therapies for burning mouth disorder may be best managed by appropriate specialist or the patient's physician due to the protracted nature of this therapy.

> **Rx:** Clonazepam (Klonopin) tabs 0.5 mg.
> Disp: 100 tabs.
> Sig: Take half to one tab three times daily and then adjust the dose after 3-day intervals. The patient should not be titrated to a dosage of greater than 2.0 mg daily.

> **Rx:** Amitriptyline (Elavil) tabs 25 mg.
> Disp: 50 tabs.
> Sig: Take 1 tab at bedtime for 1 week and then 2 tabs hs. Increase to 3 tabs hs after 2 weeks and maintain at that dosage or titrate as appropriate.

> **Rx:** Chlordiazepoxide (Librium) tabs 5 mg.
> Disp: 50 tabs.
> Sig: Take 1 or 2 tabs three times daily.

> **Rx:** Alprazolam (Xanax) tabs 0.25 mg.
> Disp: 50 tabs.
> Sig: Take 1 tab three times daily.

> **Rx:** Diazepam (Valium) tabs 2 mg.
> Disp: 50 tabs.
> Sig: Take 1 or 2 tabs three times daily. The dosage should be adjusted according to the individual response of the patient. Anticipated side effects are dry mouth and morning drowsiness.

The rationale for the use of tricyclic antidepressant medications and other psychotropic drugs should be thoroughly explained to the patient, and the patient's physician should be made aware of the therapy. These medications have a potential for addiction and dependency.

> **Rx:** Tabasco sauce (capsaicin) (OTC).
> Disp: 1 btl.
> Sig: Place one part Tabasco sauce in 2 to 4 parts of water. Rinse with 1 tsp (5 mL) for 1 min four times daily and expectorate.

> **Rx:** Capsaicin (Zostrix) crm 0.025% (OTC).
> Disp: 1 tube.
> Sig: Apply sparingly to affected site(s) four times daily. Wash hands after each application and do not use near the eyes.

Topical capsaicin may serve to improve the burning sensation in some individuals. As with topical capsaicin, an increase in discomfort for a 2- to 3-week period should be anticipated.

ADDITIONAL READINGS

Gorsky M, Silverman S Jr, Chinn H. Clinical characteristics and management outcome in the burning mouth syndrome. Oral Surg Oral Med Oral Pathol 1991;72:192–5.

Grushka M, Epstein J, Mott P. An open-label, dose escalation pilot study of the effect of clonazepam in burning mouth syndrome. Oral Surg Oral Med Oral Pathol Oral Radiol Endod 1998;86:557–61.

Lamey PJ. Burning mouth syndrome. Dermatol Clin 1996;14:339–54.

Lamey PJ, Lamb AB. Lip component of burning mouth syndrome. Oral Surg Oral Med Oral Pathol Oral Radiol Endod 1994;78:590–3.

Ship JA, Grushka M, Lipton JA, et al. Burning mouth syndrome: an update. J Am Dent Assoc 1995; 126:842–53.

2

CANDIDOSIS

ETIOLOGY

Candida albicans is a yeast-like fungus. It is an opportunistic organism that tends to proliferate with the use of broad-spectrum antibiotics, corticosteroids, medications that reduce salivary flow, and cytotoxic agents. Conditions that contribute to this disease include xerostomia, uncontrolled diabetes mellitus, anemia, poor oral hygiene, prolonged use of prosthetic oral appliances, and suppression of the immune system, such as human immunodeficiency virus (HIV) infection, or as a side effect of many medications, including steroid inhalants. Antibiotics may shift the microflora and allow overgrowth of *Candida*. It is important to determine predisposing factors prior to initiating therapy.

CLINICAL DESCRIPTION

This disease is characterized by soft, white, slightly elevated plaques that usually can be wiped away (pseudomembranous form), generalized erythematous sensitive areas (erythematous form), or confluent white areas that cannot be wiped away (hyperplastic form). Angular cheilitis, which is also described in this monograph, is frequently associated (Figure 2-1).

RATIONALE FOR TREATMENT

The rationale for the treatment of candidosis is to reestablish a normal balance of oral flora and improve oral hygiene. The disinfection of all removable oral prostheses with antifungal denture-soaking solutions and the application of antifungal agents on the tissue-contacting surfaces is necessary to remove a potential source of fungal reinfection.

Medication should be continued for a few days after disappearance of clinical signs to prevent immediate recurrence. However, several contributing authors suggest that it is advisable to empirically treat candidosis for a 10- to 14-day period. Identification and correction of contributing factors will minimize recurrence.

It is important that salivation be within normal limits. Many medications and systemic conditions, including immunosuppression, will decrease salivary flow, thereby predisposing the patient to candidosis. Increasing oral moisture by using sugarless gum or candy, mouthrinses without alcohol, or sialogogues, such as pilocarpine

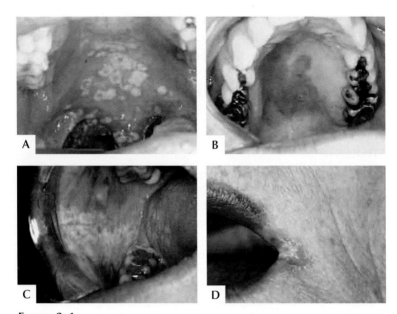

FIGURE 2-1

Clinical types of candidosis. *A,* Pseudomembranous form; *B,* erythematous form; *C,* hyperplastic form; *D,* angular cheilitis.

or cevimeline, is often an important adjunctive measure when managing candidosis (see Chapter 18, "Xerostomia [Reduced Salivary Flow and Dry Mouth]").

TOPICAL ANTIFUNGAL AGENTS

Rx: Clotrimazole (Mycelex) troches 10 mg.
Disp: 70 troches.
Sig: Let 1 troche dissolve in mouth five times daily. Do not chew.

Rx: Mycostatin pastilles 200,000 U.
Disp: 70 pastilles.
Sig: Let 1 pastille dissolve in mouth five times daily. Do not chew.

Rx: Nystatin vaginal suppositories 100,000 U.
Disp: 40 suppositories.
Sig: Let 1 suppository dissolve in the mouth four times daily. Do not rinse for 30 min.

If there is concern about the sugar content of the nystatin pastilles and clotrimazole troches, vaginal tabs/suppositories can be substituted (100–200 mg once or twice daily).

Troches/pastilles may not be well tolerated when the patient has a dry mouth because of the inability to dissolve this dosage form. Consider a course of systemic antifungal therapy.

> **Rx:** Nystatin oint.
> Disp: 15 g tube.
> Sig: Apply a thin coat to the inner surface of the denture and to the affected area after meals.

> **Rx:** Ketoconazole (Nizoral) crm 2%.
> Disp: 15 g tube.
> Sig: Apply a thin coat to the inner surface of the denture and to the affected area after meals.

> **Rx:** Clotrimazole (Gyne-Lotrimin, Mycelex-G vaginal crm 1% [OTC]).
> Disp: One tube.
> Sig: Apply a thin layer to the tissue side of the denture and/or to infected oral mucosa four times daily.

> **Rx:** Miconazole (Monistat 7) nitrate vaginal crm 2% (OTC).
> Disp: One tube.
> Sig: Apply thin layer to tissue side of denture and/or to infected oral mucosa four times daily.

Although some contributing authors disagree with the use of vaginal creams intraorally, their efficacy has been observed clinically in selected cases where other topical antifungal agents have failed.

Creams and ointments are ideal for treating patients wearing complete or partial dentures. Application of an antifungal cream or ointment to the tissue-bearing surfaces of a denture serves to localize the medication to the affected soft tissues while simultaneously treating the denture. Patients must be reminded to remove their prostheses prior to going to bed. They should be instructed to apply the cream or ointment directly to the oral soft tissues at bedtime while cleaning their denture in a commercially available denture cleanser.

A few drops of nystatin oral suspension can be added to the water used for soaking acrylic prostheses. However, most commercially available denture cleansers have some degree of antifungal activity. Dentures may be soaked in a sodium hypochlorite solution (1 tsp of sodium hypochlorite in a denture cup of water) for 15 min and thoroughly rinsed for at least 2 min under running water (long-term soaking of dentures in even a mild bleach solution will fade the pigment in the denture acrylic). Chlorhexidine gluconate and Listerine both exhibit antifungal activity.

> **Rx:** Nystatin (Mycostatin, Nilstat) oral suspension 100,000 U/mL.
> Disp: 240 mL.
> Sig: Rinse with 5 mL four times daily for 3 min by the clock and expectorate.

This is especially good for use in children because liquids are well tolerated and this medication is not toxic. If swallowed, less than 5% of this medication is absorbed systemically. This medication is of limited usefulness in the adult patient. Because of the high-sugar content, good oral hygiene must be reinforced.

SYSTEMIC ANTIFUNGAL AGENTS

Ketoconazole (Nizoral) and fluconazole (Diflucan) are effective and well-tolerated systemic drugs for mucocutaneous and oropharyngeal candidosis. They should be used with caution in patients with impaired liver function (a history of alcoholism or hepatitis). Liver function tests should be conducted periodically and/or monitored by the patient's physician when ketoconazole is prescribed for an extended period. Diminishing response over time with fluconazole may indicate development of fungal resistance or the need to temporarily increase the medication dosage.

> **Rx:** Ketoconazole (Nizoral) tabs 200 mg.
> Disp: 14 tabs.
> Sig: Take 1 tab daily with a meal or orange juice. Do not take together with buffered medications or with gastric acid blockers.

> **Rx:** Fluconazole (Diflucan) tabs 100 mg.
> Disp: 15 tabs.
> Sig: Take 2 tabs stat and then 1 tab daily until gone.

Ketaconazole and fluconazole are potent inhibitors of cytochrome P-450 isoenzymes. These antifungal medications can significantly inhibit the hepatic metabolism of medications such as antihistamines, cholesterol-lowering medications, antihypertensive medications, warfarin compounds, and antiasthmatic medications that are primarily metabolized by this liver isoenzyme system. Toxic drug interactions have been reported with both ketaconazole and fluconazole; be sure to check appropriate pharmacology references.

ADDITIONAL READINGS

Allen CM. Diagnosing and managing oral candidiasis. J Am Dent Assoc 1992;123:77–82.

Epstein JB. Antifungal therapy in oropharyngeal mycotic infections. Oral Surg Oral Med Oral Pathol 1990;69:32–41.

Fotos PG, Lilly JP. Clinical management of oral and perioral candidosis. Dermatol Clin 1996;14:273–80.

Hersh EV, Moore PA. Drug interactions in dentistry. J Am Dent Assoc 2004;135:298–311.

Lucatorto FM, Francker C, Hardy WD, et al. Treatment of refractory oral candidiasis with fluconazole: a case report. Oral Surg Oral Med Oral Pathol 1991;71:42–4.

Muzyka BC, Glick M. A review of oral fungal infections and appropriate therapy. J Am Dent Assoc 1995;126:63–72.

Scully C, El Kabir M, Samaranayake LP. Candida and oral candidosis: a review. Crit Rev Oral Biol Med 1994;5:125–57.

Siegel MA. Strategies for management of commonly encountered oral mucosal disorders. J Calif Dent Assoc 1999;27:210–27.

3

CHAPPED/CRACKED LIPS

ETIOLOGY

Alternate wetting and drying of the lip surface result in inflammation and possible secondary infection.

CLINICAL DESCRIPTION

The surface of the vermilion border is rough and peeling and may be ulcerated with crusting (Figure 3-1).

RATIONALE FOR TREATMENT

To interrupt the irritating factors and allow healing.

Rx: Oral Balance Moisturizing Gel (OTC).
Disp: 42 g tube.
Sig: Apply to lips whenever necessary.

Rx: Nystatin–triamcinolone acetonide (Mycolog II, Mytrex) oint.
Disp: 15 g tube.
Sig: Apply to lips after each meal and at bedtime.

Rx: Betamethasone valerate (Valisone) oint 0.1%.
Disp: 15 g tube.
Sig: Apply to lips after meals and at bedtime.

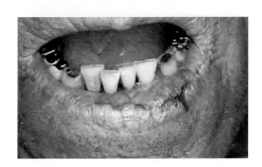

FIGURE 3-1

Severely chapped lips in a patient sensitive to lipstick.

> **Rx:** Triamcinolone acetonide (Kenalog) 0.1%.
> Disp: 15 g tube.
> Sig: Apply to lips after meals and at bedtime.

Some contributing authors suggest that three times daily application of these treatments is sufficient.

Prolonged use of corticosteroids (greater than 2 wk) should be done cautiously to minimize the potential for side effects.

For maintenance, OTC lip care products such as Oral Balance, unflavored Chapstick, Vaseline, lanolin, or cocoa butter may be considered moisturizers. Avoid products containing desiccants, such as phenol or alcohol.

If the lesion(s) does not resolve with treatment, consider a biopsy to rule out dysplasia or malignant actinic changes.

4

CHEILITIS/CHEILOSIS (ACTINIC, SOLAR)

ETIOLOGY

Prolonged exposure to sunlight results in irreversible degenerative changes in the vermilion zone of the lips.

CLINICAL DESCRIPTION

The normal red translucent vermilion zone with regular vertical fissuring of a smooth surface is replaced by a white flat surface or an irregular scaly surface that may exhibit periodic ulceration (Figure 4-1).

RATIONALE FOR TREATMENT

Elimination of exposure to UV light. Education of patient regarding malignant potential because degenerative changes may progress to malignancy.

> **Rx:** PreSun 15 lip gel (OTC).
> Disp: 15 oz.
> Sig: Apply to lips 1 h before sun exposure and every hour thereafter.

Several OTC sunscreen preparations are available (eg, PreSun 15 lotion and lip gel). For those patients allergic to PABA, non-PABA sunscreens should be suggested. For patients who have had a history of a lip malignancy, a zinc oxide product should be used.

When the lesion persists, a biopsy is required to rule out dysplasia, carcinoma in situ, or squamous cell carcinoma.

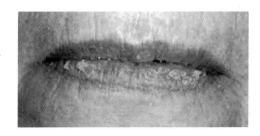

FIGURE 4-1
Sun-induced damage of the lower lip that should be managed to rule out malignant change. Note the indistinct margin between the skin and the vermilion border.

5

CHEILITIS/CHEILOSIS (ANGULAR)

ETIOLOGY

Fissured lesions in the corners of the mouth are caused by a mixed infection of the microorganisms *Candida albicans*, staphylococci, and streptococci. Predisposing factors include excessive licking, drooling, a decrease in the intermaxillary space, anemia, vitamin deficiency immunosuppression, and an extension of oral infections.

CLINICAL DESCRIPTION

The commissures may appear wrinkled, red and fissured, cracked or crusted (Figure 5-1).

RATIONALE FOR TREATMENT

Identification and correction of predisposing factors, elimination of primary and secondary infections, eradication of inflammation.

Rx: Nystatin–triamcinolone acetonide (Mycolog II, Mytrex) oint.
Disp: 15 g tube.
Sig: Apply to affected area after meals and at bedtime.

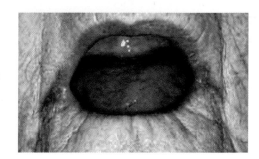

FIGURE 5-1

Cracking, erythema, and pseudomembrane formation of the labial commissures bilaterally in a patient with angular cheilitis.

Rx: Polymyxin B/Bacitracin (Polysporin) oint (OTC).
Disp: 15 g tube.
Sig: Apply to affected areas after meals and at bedtime.

Rx: Clotrimazole–betamethasone dipropionate (Lotrisone) crm.
Disp: 15 g tube.
Sig: Apply to affected area after each meal and at bedtime.

Rx: Hydrocortisone-iodoquinol (Vytone) crm 1%.
Disp: 15 g tube.
Sig: Apply to affected area after each meal and at bedtime.

Rx: Ketoconazole (Nizoral) crm 2%.
Disp: 15 g tube.
Sig: Apply sparingly to corners of mouth after each meal and at bedtime.

Rx: Clotrimazole (Gyne-Lotrimin, Mycelex-G) vaginal crm 1% (OTC).
Disp: One tube.
Sig: Apply sparingly to corners of mouth after each meal and at bedtime.

Rx: Miconazole (Monistat 7) nitrate vaginal crm 2% (OTC).
Disp: One tube.
Sig: Apply sparingly to corners of mouth after each meal and at bedtime.

Although some contributing authors disagree with the use of vaginal creams intraorally, their efficacy has been observed clinically in selected cases where other topical antifungal agents have failed.

6

DENTURE SORE MOUTH

ETIOLOGY

Discomfort under oral prosthetic appliances may result from combinations of candidal infections, poor denture hygiene, an occlusive syndrome, and overextension or excessive movement of the appliance. This condition may be erroneously attributed to an allergy to denture material, which is a rare occurrence. This condition may also represent a pressure neuropathy owing to advanced mandibular alveolar resorption exposing the mental foramen.

The retention and fit of the denture should be idealized, and mechanical irritation should be ruled out.

CLINICAL DESCRIPTION

The tissue covered by the appliance, especially one made of acrylic, is erythematous and smooth or granular. It may be either asymptomatic or associated with burning (Figure 6-1).

RATIONALE FOR TREATMENT

Therapy is directed toward controlling all possible etiologies and improving oral comfort. If therapy is ineffective, consider underlying systemic conditions, such as diabetes mellitus and poor nutrition.

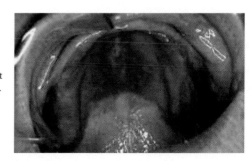

FIGURE 6-1
Denture stomatitis in a patient who did not remove his upper denture prior to bedtime.

TREATMENT

1. Institute appropriate antifungal medication (see Chapter 2, "Candidosis").
2. Improve oral and appliance hygiene. The patient may have to leave the appliance out for extended periods of time and should be instructed to leave the denture out overnight. The appliance should be soaked in a commercially available denture cleanser or soaked in a 1% sodium hypochlorite solution (1 tsp of sodium hypochlorite in a denture cup of water) for 15 min and thoroughly rinsed for at least 2 min under running water.
3. Reline, rebase, or construct a new appliance.
4. Apply an artificial saliva or oral lubricant gel, such as Laclede Oral Balance or Sage gel, to the tissue contact surface of the denture to reduce frictional trauma.

If all of the above fail to control symptoms, a biopsy or short trial of topical steroid therapy may be used to rule out contact mucositis (an allergic reaction to denture materials). If a therapeutic trial fails to resolve the condition, a biopsy should be performed to establish the diagnosis. If the patient's differential diagnosis includes any condition that may be premalignant or malignant, a biopsy should be immediately procured to determine the definitive diagnosis for the lesion.

7

ERYTHEMA MULTIFORME

ETIOLOGY

Erythema multiforme is believed to be an allergic condition. In many patients erythema multiforme seems to be an autoimmune condition because an antigen cannot be identified. It may occur at any age. Drug reactions to medications such as penicillin and sulfonamides may play a role in some cases. It has been observed in a limited number of patients who develop oral erythema multiforme that a herpetic infection occurred immediately prior to the onset of clinical signs.

CLINICAL DESCRIPTION

Signs of erythema multiforme include "blood-crusted" lips, "targetoid" or "bull's-eye" skin lesions, and a nonspecific mucosal slough. The name multiforme is used because its appearance may take multiple different forms (Figures 7-1 to 7-3). A severe form of erythema multiforme is called Stevens Johnson syndrome or erythema multiforme major. Erythema multiforme as a skin disease occurs most frequently due to an allergic reaction. This condition may occur chronically or periodically in cycles.

RATIONALE FOR TREATMENT

Treatment is primarily anti-inflammatory in nature. Steroids are initiated and then tapered.

Due to the possible relationship of erythema multiforme with herpes simplex virus, suppressive antiviral therapy may be necessary prior to initiation of steroid therapy. Patients should be carefully questioned about a previous history of recurrent herpetic infections as well as prodromal symptoms that might have preceded the onset of the erythema multiforme.

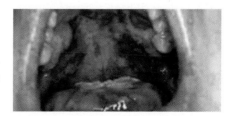

FIGURE 7-1

Palatal lesions of erythema multiforme. Note the generalized distribution and irregular borders of the lesions.

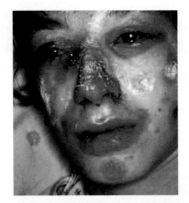

FIGURE 7-2

Erythema multiforme major (Stevens Johnson syndrome). Note the bloodshot eyes, blood-crusted lips, and targetoid skin lesions (chin).

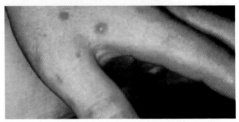

FIGURE 7-3

"Bull's-eye" or targetoid skin lesions (hand) of erythema multiforme.

Dosing must be titrated to specific situations.

STEROID THERAPY

Rx: Prednisone tablets 10 mg.
Disp: 100 tablets.
Sig: Take 6 tablets in the morning until lesions recede, then decrease by 1 tablet on each successive day. Do not exceed 14 days of therapy. If therapy exceeds 14 days, steroids should be tapered.

SUPPRESSIVE ANTIVIRAL THERAPY

Rx: Acyclovir (Zovirax), 400 mg capsules.
Disp: Sufficient quantity.
Sig: Take 1 tablet 2 times daily.

Rx: Valacyclovir (Valtrex), 500 mg caplets.
Disp: Sufficient quantity.
Sig: Take 1 or 2 caplet(s) daily.

ADDITIONAL READING

Siegel MA, Balciunas BA. Oral presentation and management of vesiculobullous disorders. Semin Dermatol 1994;13:78–86.

8

GEOGRAPHIC TONGUE (BENIGN MIGRATORY GLOSSITIS, ERYTHEMA MIGRANS)

ETIOLOGY

The etiology is unknown. Since its histologic appearance is similar to psoriasis, some have associated it with psoriasis. This may be purely coincidental. Oral lesions should not be associated with psoriasis if there are no cutaneous signs of this disorder. It has also been associated with Reiter's syndrome and generalized atopy.

CLINICAL DESCRIPTION

A benign inflammatory condition caused by desquamation of superficial keratin and filiform papillae. It is characterized by both red, denuded, irregularly shaped patches of the tongue dorsum and lateral borders surrounded by a raised, white-yellow border (Figures 8-1 and 8-2).

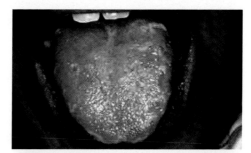

FIGURE 8-1
Geographic tongue of the tongue dorsum.

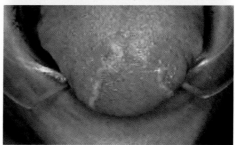

FIGURE 8-2
Close-up of geographic tongue of the tongue tip. Note the white, raised, irregular lesion border with central erythema and atrophy of the filiform lingual papillae.

RATIONALE FOR TREATMENT

Generally, no treatment is necessary because most patients are asymptomatic. When symptoms are present, they may be associated with secondary infection with *Candida albicans* (see "Supportive Care, page x"). Topical steroids, especially in combination with topical antifungal agents, are the treatment modality of choice. Patients must be told that this condition does not suggest a more serious disease and is not contagious. In most cases, biopsy is not indicated because of the pathognomonic clinical appearance. Some clinicians mix topical steroid ointments with equal parts of Orabase B paste to promote adhesion and prolong contact of the medication with the lesion being treated.

> **Rx:** Nystatin–triamcinolone acetonide (Mycolog II, Mytrex) oint.
> Disp: 15 g tube.
> Sig: Apply to affected area after each meal and at bedtime.

> **Rx:** Clotrimazole–betamethasone dipropionate (Lotrisone) crm.
> Disp: 15 g tube.
> Sig: Apply to affected area after each meal and at bedtime.

> **Rx:** Betamethasone valerate (Valisone) oint, 0.1%.
> Disp: 15 g tube.
> Sig: Apply to affected areas after meals and at bedtime.

> **Rx:** Nystatin oint.
> Disp: 15 g tube.
> Sig: Apply to affected areas after meals and at bedtime.

9

GINGIVAL OVERGROWTH

ETIOLOGY

Antiepileptic medications such as phenytoin sodium (Dilantin), calcium channel blocking agents (eg, nifedipine, diltiazem, verapamil), and cyclosporine are drugs known to predispose some patients to gingival overgrowth, especially those with poor oral hygiene practices. Poor oral hygiene, blood dyscrasias, and hereditary fibromatosis should be ruled out by clinical history, family history, and laboratory tests.

CLINICAL DESCRIPTION

The gingival tissues, especially in the anterior region, are dense, resilient, nontender, and enlarged but essentially of normal color (Figure 9-1).

RATIONALE FOR TREATMENT

Local factors such as plaque and calculus accumulation contribute to secondary inflammation and the hyperplastic process. This, in turn, further interferes with plaque control. Specific drugs tend to deplete serum folic acid levels, which may result in compromised tissue integrity.

TREATMENT

- Meticulous plaque control.
- Gingivoplasty or gingivectomy when indicated and only after oral hygiene is optimal.

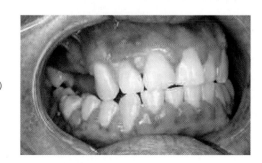

FIGURE 9-1
Drug-induced (cyclosporine) gingival overgrowth.

- When possible, replace calcium channel blockers, cyclosporine, or other implicated medications in consultation with the patient's physician.
- Test for serum folate level and supplement folic acid if necessary.
- Folic acid oral rinse.

> **Rx:** Folic acid oral rinse 1 mg/mL.
> Disp: 16 oz.
> Sig: Rinse with 1 tsp (5 mL) for 2 min twice daily and expectorate.

> **Rx:** Chlorhexidine gluconate (Peridex, PerioGard) oral rinse 0.12%.
> Disp: 473 mL (16 oz).
> Sig: Rinse with 15 mL twice for 30 seconds and spit out. Avoid rinsing or eating for 30 min following treatment. Rinse after breakfast and at bedtime.

When testing for serum folate level, it is judicious to also check for the vitamin B_{12} level because a vitamin B_{12} deficiency can be masked by the patient's use of folic acid supplement.

ADDITIONAL READINGS

Brown RS, Beaver WT, Bottomley WK. On the mechanism of drug-induced gingival hyperplasia. J Oral Pathol Med 1991;20:201–9.

Brown RS, Sein P, Corio R, Bottomley WK. Nitrendipine-induced gingival hyperplasia. Oral Surg Oral Med Oral Pathol 1990;70:593–6.

Brunet L, Miranda J, Farre M, et al. Gingival enlargement induced by drugs. Drug Saf 1996;15:219–31.

Harel-Raviv M, Eckler M, Lalani K, et al. Nifedipine-induced gingival hyperplasia: a comprehensive review and analysis. Oral Surg Oral Med Oral Pathol Oral Radiol Endod 1995;79:715–22.

10

HERPETIC GINGIVOSTOMATITIS (PRIMARY HERPES)

ETIOLOGY

Infection with HSV produces a disease that has a primary acute phase and a secondary or recurrent phase. Primary herpetic gingivostomatitis is a transmissible infection with HSV, usually type I or, less commonly, type II.

CLINICAL DESCRIPTION

Clear or yellowish vesicles develop intra- and extraorally. These rupture within hours and form shallow, painful ulcers. The gingivae are often red, enlarged, and painful (Figure 10-1). The patient may have systemic signs and symptoms, including regional lymphadenitis, fever, and malaise. Usually, it is self-limiting, with resolution in 10 to 14 days.

RATIONALE FOR TREATMENT

Treatment should focus on early intervention with antiviral agents and relieving symptoms, preventing secondary infection, and supporting general health. Supportive therapy includes forced fluids, protein, vitamin and mineral food supplements, and rest.

Systemic antiviral medications appear to be more effective if administered within the first 2 days of onset of symptoms. Topical steroid medications must be avoided because they tend to permit spread of the viral infection on mucous membranes, particularly ocular lesions. Patients should be cautioned to avoid

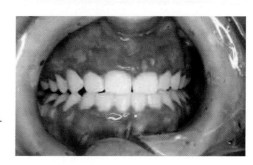

FIGURE 10-1

Primary herpetic gingivostomatitis in a child. Note the generalized erythema and edema of the gingival papillae.

touching the herpetic lesions and then touching the eye, genital, or other body areas because of the possibility of self-inoculation.

TOPICAL ANESTHETICS AND COATING AGENTS

Rx: Diphenhydramine (Children's Benadryl) elix 12.5 mg/5 mL (OTC) 4 oz mixed with Kaopectate or Maalox (OTC) 4 oz (to make a 50% mixture by volume).
Disp: 8 oz.
Sig: Rinse with 1 tsp (5 mL) every 2 h and spit out.

Rx: Diphenhydramine (Children's Benadryl) elix 12.5 mg/5 mL (OTC).
Disp: 4 oz btl.
Sig: Rinse with 1 tsp (5 mL) for 2 min every 2 h and before each meal and spit out.

Rx: Dyclonine HCl throat loz (Sucrets) (OTC).
Disp: 1 package.
Sig: Dissolve slowly in mouth every 2 h as necessary. Do not exceed 10 lozenges per day.

When topical anesthetics are used, patients should be cautioned concerning a reduced gag reflex and the need for caution while eating and drinking to avoid possible airway compromise. Allergies are rare but may occur.

SYSTEMIC ANTIVIRAL THERAPY

Acyclovir oral capsules may relieve and decrease the duration of symptoms. Acyclovir oral capsules must be initiated during the viral prodromal stage or this therapy will be ineffective.

Rx: Acyclovir (Zovirax) caps 200 mg.
Disp: 35 caps.
Sig: Take 2 caps three times daily for 7 days.

The current FDA recommendation is that systemic acyclovir be used to treat oral herpes infection only for immunocompromised patients.

Rx: Valacyclovir (Valtrex) caplets 500 mg.
Disp: 20 caplets.
Sig: Take 2 caplets twice daily for 5 days.

Based on CDC recommendation for management of primary genital herpes infection.

NUTRITIONAL SUPPLEMENTS

Rx: Meritene (protein, vitamin, mineral food supplement) (OTC).
Disp: 1 lb can (plain, vanilla, chocolate, and eggnog flavors).
Sig: Take three servings daily. Prepare as indicated on the label. Serve cold.

Rx: Ensure Plus (P-V-M Food Supplement) (OTC).
Disp: Twenty cans.
Sig: Three to five cans in divided doses throughout the day as tolerated. Serve cold.

Analgesics

Rx: Acetaminophen tablets 325 mg (OTC).
Disp: 1 btl.
Sig: Take two tabs every 4 to 6 h when necessary for pain and fever. Do not exceed 4 g per 24 h period.

FOR MODERATE TO SEVERE PAIN

Rx: Acetaminophen 300 mg with codeine 30 mg (Tylenol No. 3).
Disp: 20 tabs.
Sig: Take 1 or 2 tabs four times daily for pain.

If the patient chooses to take only one tab of Tylenol No. 3 (30 mg of codeine), the patient should be instructed to take one regular-strength acetaminophen tab (Tylenol [OTC]) to ensure the administration of the recommended strength of acetaminophen.

11

HERPES SIMPLEX RECURRENT (OROFACIAL)

ETIOLOGY

Reactivation of virus from latency in sensory ganglion of the trigeminal nerve. Precipitating factors include fever, stress, exposure to sunlight, trauma, and hormonal alterations.

CLINICAL DESCRIPTION

Intraoral*—single or small clusters of vesicles that quickly rupture, forming painful ulcers. The lesions usually occur on the keratinized tissue of the hard palate and gingiva at or near the sites of the original infection (Figure 11-1).

Labialis*—clusters of vesicles on the lips and perioral region that rupture within hours and then crust (Figure 11-2).

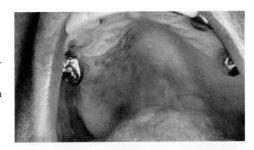

FIGURE 11-1
Recurrent intraoral herpes following a dental appointment. Note the localized distribution of the superficial lesions.

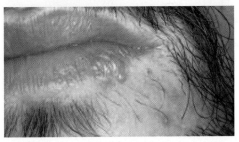

FIGURE 11-2
Recurrent herpes labialis. Note fluid-filled vesicles.

---

*In immunocompromised patients, herpes simplex virus lesions can occur on any mucosal surface and may have atypical appearances.

RATIONALE FOR TREATMENT

Treatment should be initiated as early as possible in the prodromal stage with the objective of reducing the duration and symptoms of the lesion.

Antiviral medications prophylactically as well as therapeutically may be considered when episodes are frequent (greater than six per year). Recurrent herpetic episodes interfere with daily function and nutrition. The current recommendation from the Food and Drug Administration is that systemic acyclovir be used to treat oral herpes only for immunocompromised patients. Valacyclovir has been approved for the prevention and management of oral recurrent herpes simplex infections.

PREVENTION

> **Rx:** PreSun 15 sunscreen lotion (OTC).
> Disp: 4 fl oz.
> Sig: Apply to susceptible area 1 hour before sun exposure and every hour thereafter.

> **Rx:** PreSun 15 lip gel (OTC).
> Disp: 15 oz.
> Sig: Apply to lips 1 hour before sun exposure and every hour thereafter.

If a recurrence on the lips is usually precipitated by exposure to sunlight, the lesion may be prevented by the application to the area of a sunscreen with a high skin protection factor (SPF 15 or higher).

TOPICAL ANTIVIRAL AGENTS

Topical antiviral medications are most effective when initiated as early in the course of the episode as possible. Patients should be instructed to dab on the medication as soon as prodromal symptoms are felt. These medications should be dabbed on, not rubbed in, to minimize mechanical trauma to the lesions. Patients should be instructed to apply the antiviral agent with a cotton-tip applicator.

> **Rx:** Penciclovir (Denavir) cream 1%.
> Disp: 2 g tube.
> Sig: Dab on lesion every 2 hours during waking hours, for 4 days beginning when symptoms first occur.

> **Rx:** Docosanol (Abreva) cream (OTC).
> Disp: 2 g tube.
> Sig: Dab on lesion 5 times daily during waking hours, for 4 days beginning when symptoms first occur.

SYSTEMIC ANTIVIRAL THERAPY

Systemic antiviral therapy is most effective when initiated as early in the course of the episode as possible. Patients should be instructed to take the systemic medication exactly as directed as soon as prodromal symptoms are felt. Total dosing is limited to 1 day.

> **Rx:** Valacyclovir (Valtrex) caplets 500 mg.
> Disp: 8 caplets.
> Sig: Take 4 caplets as soon as prodromal symptoms are recognized and then 4 caplets 12 hours later.

ADDITIONAL READINGS

Eisen D. The clinical characteristics of intraoral herpes simplex virus infection in 52 immuno-competent patients. Oral Surg Oral Med Oral Pathol Oral Radiol Endod 1998;86:432–7.

Greenberg MS. Herpes virus infection. Dent Clin North Am 1996;40:359–68.

Higgins CR, Schorsield JK, Tatnall FM, et al. Natural history, management and complications of herpes labialis. J Virol 1993; Suppl 1:22–6.

Miller CS. Herpes simplex virus and human papillomavirus infection of the oral cavity. Semin Dermatol 1994;13:108–17.

Poland JM. Current therapeutic management of recurrent herpes labialis. Gen Dent 1994;42:46–50.

Pope L, Marcelletti J, Katz L, et al. The anti-herpes simplex virus activity of n-docosanol includes inhibition of the viral entry process. Antiviral Res 1998;40:85–94.

Raborn GW, Chan KS, Grace M. Treatment modalities and medication recommended by health care professionals for treating recurrent herpes labialis. J Am Dent Assoc 2004;135:48–54.

Raborn GW, Martel AY, Lassonde M, et al. Effective treatment of herpes simplex labialis with penciclovir cream. J Am Dent Assoc 2002;133:303–9.

Scully C. Orofacial herpes simplex virus infections: current concepts in the epidemiology, pathogenesis, and treatment, and disorders in which the virus may be implicated. Oral Surg Oral Med Oral Pathol 1989;68:701–10.

Scully C, Epstein J, Porter S, Cox M. Viruses and chronic disorders involving the human oral mucosa. Oral Surg Oral Med Oral Pathol 1991;72:537–44.

12

HERPES ZOSTER (SHINGLES)

ETIOLOGY

Herpes zoster (shingles) represents reactivation of VZV following previous infection with chickenpox. Precipitating factors include thermal, inflammatory, radiologic, and mechanical trauma, as well as immunosuppression.

CLINICAL DESCRIPTION

Usually painful segmental eruption of small vesicles that later rupture to form punctate or confluent ulcers (Figure 12-1). Acute herpes zoster follows a portion of the trigeminal nerve distribution in about 20% of the cases. It is rare in a young individual and found more commonly in the elderly patient.

RATIONALE FOR TREATMENT

Promptly initiate antiviral therapy to reduce the duration and symptoms of the lesions. Patients over 60 years of age are particularly prone to postherpetic neuralgia (PHN). In the absence of specific contraindications, consideration should be given to prescribing short-term, high-dose, corticosteroid prophylaxis for PHN in conjunction with oral antiviral therapy.

> **Rx:** Acyclovir (Zovirax) caps 800 mg.
> Disp: 35 caps.
> Sig: Take 1 caps five times daily for 7 days.

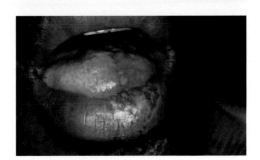

FIGURE 12-1
Herpes zoster of the skin, left lower lip, and tongue. Note that the lesions are strictly limited by the midline.

Rx: Valacyclovir (Valtrex) caplets 500 mg.
Disp: 50 caplets.
Sig: Take 2 caplets three times daily for 7 days.

ADDITIONAL READINGS

Eisen D. The clinical characteristics of intraoral herpes simplex virus infection in 52 immuno-competent patients. Oral Surg Oral Med Oral Pathol Oral Radiol Endod 1998;86:432–7.

Greenberg MS. Herpes virus infection. Dent Clin North Am 1996;40:359–68.

Higgins CR, Schorsield JK, Tatnall FM, et al. Natural history, management and complications of herpes labialis. J Virol 1993;Suppl 1:22–6.

Miller CS. Herpes simplex virus and human papillomavirus infection of the oral cavity. Semin Dermatol 1994;13:108–17.

Poland JM. Current therapeutic management of recurrent herpes labialis. Gen Dent 1994;42:46–50.

Pope L, Marcelletti J, Katz L, et al. The anti-herpes simplex virus activity of n-docosanol includes inhibition of the viral entry process. Antiviral Res 1998;40:85–94.

Raborn GW, Chan KS, Grace M. Treatment modalities and medication recommended by health care professionals for treating recurrent herpes labialis. J Am Dent Assoc 2004;135:48–54.

Raborn GW, Martel AY, Lassonde M, et al. Effective treatment of herpes simplex labialis with pen-ciclovir cream. J Am Dent Assoc 2002;133:303–9.

Scully C. Orofacial herpes simplex virus infections: current concepts in the epidemiology, patho-genesis, and treatment, and disorders in which the virus may be implicated. Oral Surg Oral Med Oral Pathol 1989;68:701–10.

Scully C, Epstein J, Porter S, Cox M. Viruses and chronic disorders involving the human oral mucosa. Oral Surg Oral Med Oral Pathol 1991;72:537–44.

13

LICHEN PLANUS

ETIOLOGY

It is postulated to be a chronic mucocutaneous autoimmune disorder with a genetic predisposition that may be initiated by a variety of factors, including emotional stress and hypersensitivity to drugs, dental products, or foods.

CLINICAL DESCRIPTION

Lichen planus varies in clinical appearance. Oral forms of this disorder include lacy white lines representing Wickham's striae (reticular), an erythematous form (atrophic), and an ulcerating form that is often accompanied by striae peripheral to the ulceration (ulcerative) (Figure 13-1). The lesions are commonly found

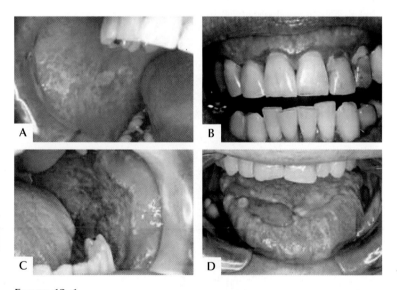

FIGURE 13-1
Clinical types of lichen planus. *A,* Reticular lichen planus. Note the striae of Wickham.
B, Atrophic lichen planus of the gingivae. Note the erythema of the free gingival margins even though the patient's plaque control appears adequate. *C,* Severe atrophic lichen planus of the left buccal mucosa. Note the atrophy of the buccal mucosa when compared with
A. D, Ulcerative lichen planus of the tongue. Note the frank ulceration of the tongue dorsum.

on the buccal mucosa, gingiva, and tongue but can be found on the lips and palate. Lichen planus lesions are chronic and may also affect the skin (Figure 13-2).

The dental and medical literature remains controversial as to whether certain forms of lichen planus transform into malignant neoplasia. Therefore, any persistent or refractory lesion(s) should be biopsied to establish a definitive diagnosis and to rule out a malignancy.

RATIONALE FOR TREATMENT

To provide oral comfort if the lesions are symptomatic. There is no known cure. Systemic and local relief with anti-inflammatory and immunosuppressant agents is indicated. Identification of any dietary component, dental product, or medication (lichenoid drug reaction) should be undertaken to ensure against a hypersensitivity reaction. Treatment or prevention of a secondary fungal infection with a systemic antifungal agent should also be considered.

Therapies with steroids and immunomodulating drugs are presented to inform the clinician that such modalities are available. Because of the potential for side effects, close collaboration with the patient's physician is recommended when these medications are prescribed. These modalities may be beyond the scope of clinical experience of general dentists, and referral to a specialist in oral medicine or to an appropriate physician may be necessary.

TOPICAL STEROIDS

> Rx: Fluocinonide (Lidex) gel 0.05%.
> Disp: 30 g tube.
> Sig: Coat the lesion with a thin film after each meal and at bedtime.

> Rx: Dexamethasone elix 0.5 mg/5 mL.
> Disp: 100 mL.
> Sig: Rinse with 1 tsp (5 mL) for 2 min four times daily and spit out. Discontinue when lesions become asymptomatic.

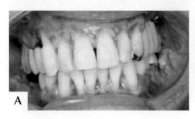 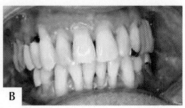

FIGURE 13-2

A 66-year-old male patient with lichen planus for a duration of 1 year. *A,* Lesions prior to treatment; *B,* lesions controlled after 10 days with systemic steroids.

Other topical steroid preparations (cream, gel ointment) include the following:

Ultrapotent

Clobetasol propionate (Temovate) 0.05%
Halobetasol propionate (Ultravate) 0.05%

Potent

Fluticasone propionate (Cutivate) 0.05%
Dexamethasone 0.5 mg/5 mL
Fluocinonide (Lidex) 0.05%

Intermediate

Aclometasone dipropionate (Aclovate) 0.05%
Betamethasone valerate (Valisone) 0.1%
Triamcinolone acetonide (Kenalog) 0.1%

Low

Hydrocortisone probutate (Pandel) 0.1%
Hydrocortisone 1%

Mixing any of the above topical steroid ointments with equal parts of Orabase B paste promotes adhesion and prolongs contact of the medication with the lesion being treated.

Prolonged use of topical steroids (greater than 2 weeks continuous use) may result in mucosal atrophy and secondary candidosis and increase the potential of systemic absorption. It may be necessary to prescribe antifungal therapy with steroids. Therapy with topical steroids, once the lichen planus is under control, should be tapered to alternate-day therapy or less depending on disease control and tendency to recur.

Oral candidosis may result from topical steroid therapy. The oral cavity should be monitored for emergence of fungal infection on patients who are placed on therapy. Prophylactic antifungal therapy should be initiated in patients with a history of fungal infections with previous steroid administration (see Chapter 2, "Candidosis").

SYSTEMIC STEROIDS AND IMMUNOSUPPRESSANTS

For severe cases,

> **Rx:** Dexamethasone elix 0.5 mg/5 mL.
> Disp: 320 mL.
> Sig: As directed in writing not to exceed 2 continuous weeks.

Directions for using dexamethasone elix:

Rinse for 1 min by the clock, four times daily, after meals and before bedtime. Do not drink or eat for 30 min after rinsing with dexamethasone elixir. Discontinue medication when lesions resolve.

- For 3 days, rinse with 1 tbsp (15 mL) four times daily and swallow. Then,
- For 3 days, rinse with 1 tsp (5 mL) four times daily and swallow. Then,
- For 3 days, rinse with 1 tsp (5 mL) four times daily and swallow every other time. Then,
- Rinse with 1 tsp (5 mL) four times daily and expectorate.

> **Rx:** Tacrolimus 0.1% oint.
> **Disp:** 30 g tube.
> **Sig:** Apply to affected site(s) twice daily as directed.

> **Rx:** Tacrolimus 0.03% oint.
> **Disp:** 30 g tube.
> **Sig:** Apply to affected site(s) twice daily as directed.

> **Rx:** Prednisone tabs 10 mg.
> **Disp:** 26 tabs.
> **Sig:** Take 4 tabs in the morning for 5 days and then decrease by 1 tab on each successive day.

> **Rx:** Prednisone tabs 5 mg.
> **Disp:** 40 tabs.
> **Sig:** Take 5 tabs in the morning for 5 days and then 5 tabs in the morning every other day until gone.

If oral discomfort recurs, the patient should return to the clinician for reevaluation.

Therapy with medications such as systemic steroids, immunosuppressants, and immunomodulators is presented to inform the clinician that such modalities have been reported effective for patients suffering from ulcerative lichen planus. Medications such as azathioprine, mycophenolate mofetil, tacrolimus, hydroxychloroquine-sulfate, acitretin, and cyclosporine are used to treat patients with severe persistent ulcerative lichen planus but should not be routinely used because of the potential for side effects. Close collaboration with the patient's physician is recommended when these medications are prescribed.

Topical tacrolimus has been associated with neoplastic disease, such as lymphoma, and, therefore, should not be used indiscriminately for long periods of time. This medication is indicated for patients who cannot tolerate or are refractory to topical or systemic steroid therapy.

All patients with lichen planus must be periodically followed for control of discomfort and to ensure against the very low risk of malignant transformation.

ADDITIONAL READINGS

Bagan JV, Ramon C, Gonzalez L, et al. Preliminary investigation of the association of oral lichen planus and hepatitis C. Oral Surg Oral Med Oral Pathol Oral Radiol Endod 1998;85:532–6.

Berkhart NW, Burker EJ, Burkes EJ, et al. Assessing the characteristics of patients with oral lichen planus. J Am Dent Assoc 1996;127:648–56.

Chainani-Wu N, Silverman S Jr, Lozada-Nur F, et al. Oral lichen planus: patient profile, disease progression and treatment responses. J Am Dent Assoc 2001;132:901–9.

Eisen DE. The evaluation of cutaneous, genital, scalp, nail, esophageal and ocular involvement in patients with oral lichen planus. Oral Surg Oral Med Oral Pathol Oral Radiol Endod 1999;88:431–6.

Epstein JB, Wan LS, Gorsky M, Zhang L. Oral lichen planus: progress in understanding its malignant potential and the implications of clinical management. Oral Surg Oral Med Oral Pathol Oral Radiol Endod 2003;96:32–7.

FDA public health advisory. Elidel (pimecrolimus) cream and Protopic (tacrolimus) ointment. March 10, 2005. Available at: http://www.fda.gov/cder/drug/advisory/elidel_protopic.htm (accessed April 1, 2005).

Gonzales-Moles MA, Morales P, Rodriguez-Archilla A, et al. Treatment of severe chronic oral erosive lesions with clobetasol propionate in aqueous solution. Oral Surg Oral Med Oral Pathol Oral Radiol Endod 2002;93:264–70.

Miles DA, Howard MM. Diagnosis and management of oral lichen planus. Dermatol Clin 1996;14:281–90.

Ostman P, Anneroth G, Skoglund A. Amalgam-associated oral lichenoid reactions. Oral Surg Oral Med Oral Pathol Oral Radiol Endod 1996;81:459–65.

Plemons JM, Rees TD, Zachariah NY. Absorption of a topical steroid and evaluation of adrenal suppression in patients with erosive lichen planus. Oral Surg Oral Med Oral Pathol 1990;69:688–93.

Silverman S Jr, Gorsky M, Lozada-Nur F, Giannotti K. A prospective study of findings and management in 214 patients with oral lichen planus. Oral Surg Oral Med Oral Pathol 1991;72:665–70.

Silverman S Jr, Gorsky M, Lozada-Nur F. A prospective follow-up study of 570 patients with oral lichen planus: persistence remission and malignant association. Oral Surg Oral Med Oral Pathol 1985;69:30–4.

van der Meij EH, Schepman KP, Smeele LE, et al. A review of the recent literature regarding malignant transformation of oral lichen planus. Oral Surg Oral Med Oral Pathol Oral Radiol Endod 1999;88:307–10.

van der Meij EH, Schepman KP, van der Waal I. The possible premalignant character of oral lichen planus and oral lichenoid lesions: a prospective study. Oral Surg Oral Med Oral Pathol Oral Radiol Endod 2003;96:164–71.

Van Dis ML, Parks ET. Prevalence of oral lichen planus in patients with diabetes mellitus. Oral Surg Oral Med Oral Pathol Oral Radiol Endod 1995;79:696–700.

Vincent SD, Fotos PG, Baker KA, Williams TP. Oral lichen planus: the clinical, historical, and therapeutic features of 100 cases. Oral Surg Oral Med Oral Pathol 1990;70:165–71.

14

MANAGEMENT OF PATIENTS RECEIVING ANTINEOPLASTIC AGENTS AND RADIATION THERAPY

ETIOLOGY

Head and neck radiation treatment of oral cancer can reduce saliva volume and composition when a major salivary gland is in the primary radiation field. Oral tissue delivery of multiple antimicrobial components of saliva, including histatins, lactoferrin, and lysozyme, is typically decreased. The balance of oral flora is then disrupted, allowing overgrowth of opportunistic organisms, such as *Candida albicans*. Advances over the past several years, including salivary gland protection during radiation dosing (via amifostine) and/or saliva stimulant (secretogogue) intervention (via pilocarpine hydrochloride or cevimeline), have helped reduce the morbidity associated with long-term salivary gland hypofunction in these patients.

Patients receiving anticholinergic medications during high-dose chemotherapy may also experience salivary compromise. However, glandular function tends to return to normal in the weeks following discontinuation of these medications.

Cytotoxic cancer therapy can also impair normal, rapidly dividing cells, including those of the oral mucosa. This can result in painful, ulcerative oral mucositis with important clinical consequences. One drug, palifermin, is approved by the FDA for reducing the severity of oral mucositis in patients with hematologic malignancies who are receiving a bone marrow transplant. Other drugs for mucositis management are in development but are not FDA approved at this time for use outside a research environment.

The information listed below is intended to assist the practicing dentist in the management of oncology patients once they are in an outpatient setting.

CLINICAL DESCRIPTION

The oral mucosa becomes red, inflamed, and/or ulcerated. The saliva may be viscous or absent (Figure 14-1).

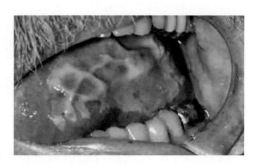

FIGURE 14-1
Radiation-induced mucositis
of the tongue.

RATIONALE FOR TREATMENT

The treatment of these patients is symptomatic and supportive and should be aimed at patient comfort and education, maintenance of proper nutrition and oral hygiene, and prevention of opportunistic infection. Frequent monitoring and close cooperation with the patient's physician are important.

All patients must have a preradiation therapy oral evaluation to eliminate any source of infection. Whenever possible, 14 days of oral healing time should be allowed prior to initiation of radiation therapy following oral surgical procedures. Oral hygiene is of paramount importance prior to, during, and after radiation therapy.

The oral discomfort may be relieved with topical anesthetics such as lidocaine HCl (Xylocaine) viscous, diphenhydramine elixir (Benadryl), and throat lozenges containing dyclonine HCl. Artificial salivas (eg, Sage Moist Plus, Moi-Stir, Salivart, Xero-lube) will reduce oral dryness. Mouth moisturizing gels such as Laclede Oral Balance gel are helpful. Nystatin and clotrimazole preparations will control fungal overgrowth. Chlorhexidine rinses help control plaque and candidosis. Fluorides are applied for caries control (dentifrices, gels, rinses).

MOUTHRINSES (SEE CHAPTER 18, "XEROSTOMIA [REDUCED SALIVARY FLOW AND DRY MOUTH]")

> **Rx:** Alkaline saline (salt/bicarbonate) mouthrinse.
> Disp: Mix ½ tsp each of salt and baking soda in 16 oz of water.
> Sig: Rinse with copious amounts at least five times daily.

Commercially available as Sage Salt & Soda Rinse.

GINGIVITIS CONTR\OL

> **Rx:** Chlorhexidine gluconate (Peridex, PerioGard) 0.12%.
> Disp: 473 mL (16 oz).
> Sig: Rinse with 15 mL twice for 30 seconds and spit out. Avoid rinsing or eating for 30 min following treatment. Rinse after breakfast and at bedtime.

In xerostomic patients, chlorhexidine gluconate should be used concurrently with artificial saliva to provide the needed protein-binding agent for efficacy and substantivity.

CARIES CONTROL (SEE CHAPTER 18)

> **Rx:** Neutral NaF gel (Thera-Flur-N) 1.1% or PreviDent 1.1%.
> Disp: 1 tube.
> Sig: Place 1 inch ribbon on toothbrush; brush for 2 min daily and expectorate. Avoid rinsing or eating for 30 min following treatment.

TOPICAL COATING AGENTS AND ANESTHETICS

> **Rx:** Sucralfate (Carafate) suspension 1 g/10 mL.
> Disp: 420 mL (14 oz).
> Sig: Rinse with 1 tsp (5 mL) every 2 h and spit out.

> **Rx:** Diphenhydramine (Children's Benadryl) elix 12.5 mg/5 mL (OTC) 4 oz mixed with Kaopectate or Maalox (OTC) 4 oz (to make a 50% mixture by volume).
> Disp: 8 oz.
> Sig: Rinse with 1 tsp (5 mL) every 2 h and spit out.

> **Rx:** Diphenhydramine (Children's Benadryl) elix 12.5 mg/5 mL (OTC).
> Disp: 4 oz btl.
> Sig: Rinse with 1 tsp (5 mL) for 2 min before each meal and expectorate.

> **Rx:** Dyclonine HCl throat lozenges (Sucrets) (OTC).
> Disp: 1 package.
> Sig: Dissolve slowly in mouth every 2 h as necessary. Do not exceed 10 lozenges per day.

When topical anesthetics are used, patients should be cautioned concerning a reduced gag reflex and the need for caution while eating and drinking to avoid possible airway compromise.

ANTIFUNGAL AGENTS

See Chapter 2, "Candidosis."

SALIVA STIMULANTS

See Chapter 18, "Xerostomia (Reduced Salivary Flow and Dry Mouth)."

15

PEMPHIGUS VULGARIS AND MUCOUS MEMBRANE PEMPHIGOID

These are relatively uncommon conditions. They should be suspected when there are chronic, multiple oral ulcerations and a history of oral and skin blisters. Often they may occur only in the mouth. Diagnosis is based on the history and the histologic and immunofluorescent characteristics of a biopsy of the primary lesion.

ETIOLOGY

Both are autoimmune diseases with autoantibodies against antigens appearing in different portions of the epithelium (mucosa). In pemphigus, the antigens are within the epithelium (desmosomes), whereas in pemphigoid, the antigens are located at the base of the epithelium in the hemidesmosomes.

CLINICAL CHARACTERISTICS

In pemphigus, the lesion may stay in one location for a long period of time with small placid bullae. The bullae may rupture, leaving an ulcer. Approximately 80 to 90% of the patients have oral lesions. In approximately two-thirds of patients, the oral manifestations are the first sign of the disease. All parts of the mouth may be involved (Figure 15-1). The bullae rupture almost immediately in the mouth but may stay intact for some time on the skin (Figure 15-2). One of the classic signs, Nikolsky's sign (blister formation induced with gentle rubbing of a normal, perilesional mucosal site), is positive in pemphigus but is not pathognomic because it has also been found positive in other disorders. Because the vesicle or bulla is intraep-

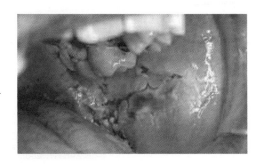

FIGURE 15-1
Pemphigus vulgaris of the buccal mucosa and hard palate. Note the extensive distribution of these superficial erosive lesions.

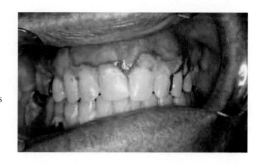

FIGURE 15-2

Mucous membrane pemphigoid of the gingivae. Note the intact blood-filled bullous lesions of the gingivae.

ithelial, it is often filled with clear fluid. Histologically, there is a cleavage (Tzanck cells, acantholytic cells) within the spinous layer of the epithelium.

In pemphigoid, the cleavage or split is beneath the epithelium, resulting in bullae that are usually blood filled. Mucous membrane pemphigoid is often limited to the oral cavity, but some patients have ocular lesions (symblepharon, ankyloblepharon) that need to be evaluated by an ophthalmologist. The gingiva is the most common oral site involved. Pemphigoid may appear clinically as a red, nonulcerated gingival lesion. Patients should be queried with regard to ocular or pharyngeal involvement.

RATIONALE FOR TREATMENT

Since both pemphigus and pemphigoid are autoimmune disorders, the primary treatment is topical or systemic steroids or other immunomodulating drugs (Figure 15-3). Pemphigus requires the use of systemic medications. Custom trays may be used to localize topical steroid medications on the gingival tissues (occlusive therapy). Because they can resemble other ulcerative-bullous diseases, a biopsy is necessary for a definitive diagnosis. Specimens should be submitted for light microscopic, immunofluorescent, and immunologic testing. Because of the potential serious nature, referral to specialists in oral medicine, dermatology, otorhinolaryngology, and ophthalmology must be considered. When eye lesions are present, an ophthalmologist must be consulted immediately to prevent blindness.

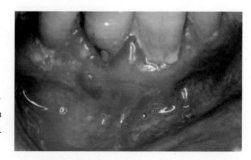

FIGURE 15-3

A 60-year-old female patient with mucous membrane pemphigoid for a duration of 1 year. *A,* Lesions prior to treatment; *B,* lesions controlled with topical steroids at bedtime only.

Therapy with medications such as systemic steroids, immunosuppressants, and immunomodulators is presented to inform the clinician that such modalities have been reported effective for patients suffering from vesiculobullous disorders such as pemphigus vulgaris and mucous membrane pemphigoid. Therapies such as dapsone, methotrexate, mycophenolate mofetil, cyclosporine, niacinamide with tetracycline, and plasmapheresis are used to treat patients with vesiculobullous disorders such as pemphigus vulgaris and mucous membrane pemphigoid but should not be routinely used because of the potential for side effects. Close collaboration with the patient's physician is recommended when these medications are prescribed.

ADDITIONAL READINGS

Ciarrocca KN, Greenberg MS. A retrospective study of the management of oral mucous membrane pemphigoid with dapsone. Oral Surg Oral Med Oral Pathol Oral Radiol Endod 1999;88:159–63.

Dayan S, Simmons RK, Ahmed AR. Contemporary issues in the diagnosis of oral pemphigoid. Oral Surg Oral Med Oral Pathol Oral Radiol Endod 1999;88:424–30.

Gonzales-Moles MA, Ruiz-Avila I, Rodriguez-Archilla A, et al. Treatment of severe erosive gingival lesions by topical application of clobetasol propionate in custom trays. Oral Surg Oral Med Oral Pathol Oral Radiol Endod 2003;95:688–92.

Gorsky M, Raviv M, Raviv E. Pemphigus vulgaris in adolescence: a case presentation and review of the literature. Oral Surg Oral Med Oral Pathol 1994;77:620–2.

Lilly JP, Spivey JD, Fotos PG. Benign mucous membrane pemphigoid with advanced periodontal involvement: diagnosis and therapy. J Periodontol 1995;66:737–41.

Lozada-Nur F, Miranda C, Miliksi R. Double-blind clinical trial of 0.05% clobetasol propionate ointment in Orabase and 0.05% fluocinonide ointment in Orabase in the treatment of patients with oral vesiculoerosive diseases. Oral Surg Oral Med Oral Pathol 1994;77:598–604.

Porter SR, Scully C, Midda M, et al. Adult linear immunoglobulin A disease manifesting as desquamative gingivitis. Oral Surg Oral Med Oral Pathol 1990;70:450–3.

Robinson JC, Lozada-Nur F, Frieden I. Oral pemphigus vulgaris: a review of the literature and a report on the management of 12 cases. Oral Surg Oral Med Oral Pathol Oral Radiol Endod 1997;84:349–55.

Siegel MA. Intraoral biopsy technique for direct immunofluorescence studies. Oral Surg Oral Med Oral Pathol 1991;72:681–4.

Siegel MA, Anhalt GJ. Direct immunofluorescence of detached gingival epithelium for diagnosis of cicatricial pemphigoid. Oral Surg Oral Med Oral Pathol 1993;75:296–302.

16

RECURRENT
APHTHOUS STOMATITIS

ETIOLOGY

An altered local immune response is the predisposing factor. Patients with frequent recurrences should be screened for diseases such as anemia, diabetes mellitus, vitamin deficiency, inflammatory bowel disease, and immunosuppression.

Precipitating factors include stress, trauma, allergies, and endocrine alterations, as well as dietary components, such as acidic foods and juices and foods that contain gluten. Inspect the oral cavity closely for sources of trauma.

CLINICAL DESCRIPTION

Minor aphthae (canker sore): < 0.5 cm, small, shallow, painful ulceration covered by a gray membrane and surrounded by a narrow erythematous halo (Figure 16-1A and 1B). They usually occur on nonkeratinized (moveable) oral mucosa. These lesions heal without scarring. Minor aphthae are the most commonly occurring lesions of recurrent aphthous stomatitis.

Major aphthae: > 0.5 cm, large, painful ulcers. Major aphthae represent a more severe form of recurrent aphthous stomatitis that may last from 6 weeks to 3 months (Figure 16-1C). Healing may result in mucosal scarring. These ulcerations may mimic other diseases, such as granulomatous or malignant lesions.

Herpetiform ulcers: crops of small, shallow, painful ulcers (Figure 16-1D). They may occur anywhere on nonkeratinized oral mucosa and resemble recurrent, intraoral herpes simplex infection clinically but are of unknown etiology.

RATIONALE FOR TREATMENT

Effective treatment involves barriers, amlexanox, cauterization, topical or systemic corticosteroids, and immunosuppressant or combination therapy when indicated. Treatment should be initiated as early in the course of the lesions as possible. Identification and elimination of precipitating factors may serve to minimize recurrent episodes. Medications such as mycophenolate mofetil, pentoxiphylline, colchicine, and thalidomide are used to treat patients with severe, persistent recurrent aphthous ulcers (RAU) but should not be routinely used.

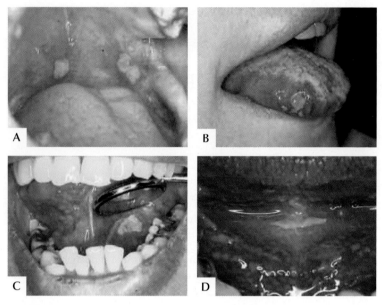

FIGURE 16-1

Clinical types of recurrent aphthous ulceration. *A,* Minor aphthous ulcerations of the tongue and soft palate. Note the round to ovoid shape of these lesions and their occurrence on nonkeratinized tissues. *B,* Minor aphthous ulceration on the lateral border of the tongue in a child. *C,* Major aphthous ulceration on the floor of the mouth. *D,* Herpetiform aphthous ulcerations of the floor of the mouth. Note that the distribution is limited to nonkeratinized mucosal tissues.

Mixing topical steroid ointments with equal parts of Orabase B paste promotes adhesion and prolongs contact of the medication with the lesion being treated.

NONSTEROIDAL TOPICAL PREPARATIONS

> **Rx:** Amlexanox oral paste 5%.
> Disp: 5 g tube.
> Sig: Dab on affected area(s) four times daily until healed.

> **Rx:** Orabase Soothe-N-Seal Protective Barrier (OTC).
> Disp: 1 package.
> Sig: Apply as per the package directions every 6 h when necessary.

Therapies with steroids and immunomodulating drugs are presented to inform the clinician that such modalities are available. Because of the potential for side effects, close collaboration with the patient's physician is recommended if these medications are prescribed. These modalities may be beyond the scope of clinical experience of general dentists, and referral to a specialist in oral medicine or to an appropriate physician may be necessary.

TOPICAL STEROIDS

Mixing topical steroid ointments with equal parts of Orabase B paste promotes adhesion and prolongs contact of the medication with the lesion being treated.

> **Rx:** Dexamethasone elix 0.5 mg/5 mL.
> Disp: 100 mL.
> Sig: Rinse with 1 tsp (5 mL) for 2 min four times daily and expectorate. Discontinue when lesions become asymptomatic.

> **Rx:** Triamcinolone acetonide (Kenalog) in Orabase 0.1%.
> Disp: 5 g tube.
> Sig: Coat the lesion with a thin film after each meal and at bedtime.

Other topical steroid preparations (cream, gel rinse, ointment) include the following:

Ultrapotent

Clobetasol propionate (Temovate) 0.05%
Halobetasol propionate (Ultravate) 0.05%

Potent

Fluticasone propionate (Cutivate) 0.05%
Dexamethasone (Decadron) 0.5 mg/5 mL
Fluocinonide (Lidex) 0.05%

Intermediate

Aclometasone dipropionate (Aclovate) 0.05%
Betamethasone valerate (Valisone) 0.1%
Triamcinolone acetonide (Kenalog) 0.1%

Low

Hydrocortisone probutate (Pandel) 0.1%
Hydrocortisone 1%

Prolonged use of topical steroids (greater than 2 weeks of continuous use) may result in mucosal atrophy and secondary candidiosis and increase the potential for systemic absorption. Their chronic use is discouraged. It may be necessary to prescribe antifungal therapy with steroids.

Oral candidosis may result from topical steroid therapy. The oral cavity should be monitored for emergence of fungal infection on patients who are placed on therapy. Prophylactic antifungal therapy should be initiated in patients with a history of fungal infections during previous steroid administration (see Chapter 2, "Candidosis").

SYSTEMIC STEROIDS AND IMMUNOSUPPRESSANTS

For severe cases,

> **Rx:** Dexamethasone elix 0.5 mg/5 mL.
> Disp: 320 mL.
> Sig: As directed in writing, not to exceed 2 continuous weeks.

Directions for using dexamethasone elixir:

Rinse for 1 min by the clock, four times daily, after meals and before bedtime. Do not drink or eat for 30 min after rinsing with dexamethasone elixir. Discontinue medication when lesions resolve.

1. For 3 days, rinse with 1 tbsp (15 mL) four times daily and swallow. Then,
2. For 3 days, rinse with 1 tsp (5 mL) four times daily and swallow. Then,
3. For 3 days, rinse with 1 tsp (5 mL) four times daily and swallow every other time. Then
4. Rinse with 1 tsp (5 mL) four times daily and expectorate.

> **Rx:** Prednisone tabs 5 mg.
> Disp: 40 tabs.
> Sig: Take 5 tabs in the morning for 5 days and then 5 tabs in the morning every other day until gone.

For very severe cases,

> **Rx:** Prednisone tabs 10 mg.
> Disp: 26 tabs.
> Sig: Take 4 tabs in the morning for 5 days and then decrease by 1 tab on each successive day until gone.

Therapy with medications such as systemic steroids, immunosuppressants, and immunomodulators is presented to inform the clinician that such modalities have been reported effective for patients suffering from severe, persistent, recurrent aphthous stomatitis. Medications such as azathioprine, pentoxiphylline, levamisole, colchicine, dapsone, and thalidomide are used to treat patients with severe, persistent recurrent aphthous stomatitis but should not be routinely used because of the potential for side effects. Close collaboration with the patient's physician is recommended when these medications are prescribed.

ADDITIONAL READINGS

Brown RS, Bottomley WK. Combination immunosuppressant and topical therapy for treatment of recurrent major aphthae. Oral Surg Oral Med Oral Pathol 1990;69:42–4.

Chandrasekhar J, Liem AA, Cox NH, Paterson AW. Oxypentifylline in the management of recurrent aphthous oral ulcers. Oral Surg Oral Med Oral Pathol Oral Radiol Endod 1999;87:564–7.

Cohen DM, Bhattacharyya I, Lydiatt WM. Recalcitrant oral ulcers caused by calcium channel blockers: diagnosis and treatment considerations. J Am Dent Assoc 1999;130:1611–8.

Khandwala A, Van Inwegen RG, Alfano MC. 5% amlexanox oral paste, a new treatment for recurrent minor aphthous ulcers. II. Pharmacokinetics and demonstration of clinical safety. Oral Surg Oral Med Oral Pathol Oral Radiol Endod 1997;83:231–8.

Kutcher MJ, Ludlow JB, Samuelson AD, et al. Evaluation of a bioadhesive device for the management of aphthous ulcers. J Am Dent Assoc 2001;132:368–76.

Lozada F, Silverman S Jr, Migliorati C. Adverse side effects associated with prednisone in the treatment of patients with oral inflammatory ulcerative diseases. J Am Dent Assoc 1984;109:269–70.

Ogura M, Morita M, Wantanabe T. A case controlled study on food intake of patients with recurrent aphthous stomatitis. Oral Surg Oral Med Oral Pathol Oral Radiol Endod 2001;91:45–9.

Porter SR, Kingsmill V, Scully C. Audit of diagnosis and investigations in patients with recurrent aphthous stomatitis. Oral Surg Oral Med Oral Pathol 1993;76:449–52.

Scully C, Azul AM, Crighton A, et al. Nicorandil can induce severe oral ulceration. Oral Surg Oral Med Oral Pathol Oral Radiol Endod 2001;91:189–93.

Ship JA. Recurrent aphthous stomatitis. Oral Surg Oral Med Oral Pathol Oral Radiol Endod 1996;81:141–7.

Siegel MA, Balciunas BA. Medication can induce severe ulcerations. J Am Dent Assoc 1991;122:75–7.

Woo SB, Sonis ST. Recurrent aphthous ulcers: a review of diagnosis and treatment. J Am Dent Assoc 1996:127:1202–13.

17

TASTE AND SMELL DISORDERS (CHEMOSENSORY DISORDERS)

ETIOLOGY

Taste acuity may be affected by medications and by neurologic and physiologic changes. Complaints of taste loss should be differentiated from alterations in flavor perception, which is primarily derived from smell. Clinical examination and diagnostic procedures may identify potential etiologic factors such as nasal sinus disease (nasal polyps), viral infection, oral candidosis, neoplasia, malnutrition, metabolic disturbances, chemical and physical trauma, drugs, and radiation sequelae. In some patients, anxiety or depression might be considered. Quantitative tests that assess salivary flow and the patient's ability to identify and discriminate odorants and taste stimuli may be useful. Laboratory studies for trace elements may be necessary to identify any existing deficiencies.

RATIONALE FOR TREATMENT

A reduction in salivary flow may concentrate electrolytes in the saliva, resulting in a salty or metallic taste (dysgeusia) (see Chapter 18, "Xerostomia [Reduced Salivary Flow and Dry Mouth]").

Several medications, including angiotensin-converting enzyme inhibitors and lithium carbonate, are known to cause taste alterations. It may be prudent to contact the patient's physician to substitute these medications when practical. Oral hygiene must be optimal because patients may compensate for changes in taste or flavor acuity by overusing sugars.

A deficiency of zinc, albeit rare, has been associated with a loss of taste (and smell) sensation. To prevent deficiency, the current recommended dietary allowance for zinc is 12 to 15 mg for adults. Additional zinc supplementation should be reserved for individuals with true deficiency states.

TO ENSURE DIETARY ALLOWANCE FOR ZINC

Rx: Z-BEC tabs (OTC).
Disp: 60 tabs.
Sig: Take 1 tab daily with food or after meals.

ADDITIONAL READINGS

Henkin RI. Drug-induced taste and smell disorders. Incidence, mechanisms and management related primarily to treatment of sensory receptor dysfunction. Drug Saf 1994;11:318–77.

Heyneman CA. Zinc deficiency and taste disorder. Ann Pharmacother 1996;30:186–7.

Mott AE, Grushka M, Sessle BJ. Diagnosis and management of taste disorders and burning mouth syndrome. Dent Clin North Am 1993;37:33–71.

Ship JA. Gustatory and olfactory considerations in general dental practice. J Am Dent Assoc 1993;124:55–61.

18

Xerostomia (Reduced Salivary Flow and Dry Mouth)

ETIOLOGY

Acute or chronic salivary flow alterations or xerostomia may result from drug therapy, mechanical blockage, dehydration, emotional stress, bacterial infection of the salivary glands, local surgery, avitaminosis, diabetes, anemia, connective tissue diseases, Sjögren's syndrome, radiation therapy, viral infections, and certain congenital disorders.

CLINICAL DESCRIPTION

The saliva may be ropey, with a film forming over the teeth. The tissue may be dry, pale or red, and atrophic. The tongue may be devoid of papillae, atrophic, fissured, and inflamed. Multiple carious lesions may be present, especially at the gingival margin and on exposed root surfaces (Figure 18-1). The quantity and the quality of saliva may be altered.

RATIONALE FOR TREATMENT

Salivary stimulation or replacement therapy to keep the mouth moist, prevention of caries and candidal infection, and palliative relief.

For patients with removable dentures, the application of an artificial saliva or oral lubricant gel to the tissue contact surface of the denture reduces frictional trauma.

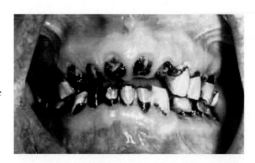

FIGURE 18-1
Severe radiation-induced xerostomia and caries. Note the atrophic appearance of the soft tissues and the extensive class V and root caries.

SALIVA SUBSTITUTES

> **Rx:** Sodium carboxymethylcellulose 0.5% aqueous solution (OTC).
> Disp: 8 fl oz.
> Sig: Use as a rinse as frequently as needed. Generic carboxymethylcellulose solutions may be prepared by a pharmacist.

Plain water in a small plastic bottle is often used with success by many xerostomic patients.

COMMERCIAL SALIVA SUBSTITUTES (OTC)

- Glandosane
- Moi-Stir
- Mouth Kote
- Roxane Saliva Substitute
- Sage Moist Plus
- Salivart
- Xero-lube
- Ask your pharmacist

COMMERCIAL ORAL MOISTURIZING GELS (OTC)

- Laclede Oral Balance
- Sage Mouth Moisturizer

Relief from oral dryness and accompanying discomfort can be achieved conservatively by

- Sipping water frequently all day long
- Letting ice melt in the mouth
- Restricting caffeine and cola intake
- Avoiding mouth rinses, drinks, and medications containing alcohol
- Avoiding tobacco products
- Humidifying the sleeping area
- Coating the lips (see Chapter 3, "Chapped/Cracked Lips")

SALIVA STIMULANTS

The use of sugar-free gum, lemon drops, or mints is a conservative method to temporarily stimulate salivary flow in patients with medication xerostomia or with salivary gland dysfunction. Patients should be cautioned against using products that contain sugar or have a low pH.

> **Rx:** Biotene chewing gum (OTC).
> Disp: 1 package.
> Sig: Chew as needed.

Owing to problems of abrasion of the mucosa under the denture and potential adhesion of the gum to the denture, use caution if the patient wears removable dentures.

> **Rx:** Pilocarpine HCl (Salagen) tabs 5 mg.
> Disp: 21 tabs.
> Sig: Take 1 tab three times daily 30 min prior to meals. Dose may be titrated to 2 tabs three times daily.

Some contributing authors recommend using 1 tab of pilocarpine four to five times daily.

> **Rx:** Cevimeline (Evoxac) caps 30 mg.
> Disp: 21 caps.
> Sig: Take 1 cap three times daily.

> **Rx:** Pilocarpine HCL sol 1 mg/mL.
> Disp: 100 mL.
> Sig: Take 1 tsp (5 mL) four times daily.

> **Rx:** Bethanechol (Urecholine) tabs 25 mg.
> Disp: 30 tab.
> Sig: Take 1 tab up to 5 times daily.

Cholinergic drugs should be prescribed in consultation with the physician-of-record or specialist owing to significant side effects. The pilocarpine and cevimeline dosage should be adjusted to increase saliva while minimizing the adverse side effects (eg, sweating, stomach upset). Patients should be warned that there is a wide range of sensitivity and that the adverse side effects may exceed the desired increased salivation; if this occurs, then the cholinergic drug should be discontinued.

CARIES PREVENTION

> **Rx:** Fluoride gel (see examples below).
> Disp: 1 tube.
> Sig: Place a 1-inch ribbon in a custom tray; apply for 5 min daily. Avoid rinsing or eating for 30 min following treatment.

> **Rx:** Fluoride gel (see examples below).
> Disp: 1 tube.
> Sig: Place a 1-inch ribbon on a toothbrush; brush for 2 min daily and expectorate. Avoid rinsing or eating for 30 min following treatment.

TABLE 18-1. FLUORIDE GELS	
0.4% Stannous Fluoride	*1.1% Neutral or Acidulated Sodium Fluoride*
Alpha-Dent	Control Rx
Easy-Gel	Karigel-N
Florentine II	Oral-B Neutracare
Gel-Kam	PreviDent gel
Gel-Tin	PreviDent 5000 Plus
Kids Choice	ProDenTx 1.1% Plus
Omnii Gel	Thera-Flur-N
Oral-B Stop	
Perfect Choice	
Periocheck Oral Med	
Plak Smacker	
Schein Home Care	
Superdent	

Rx: PreviDent 1.1% gel.
Disp: 1 tube.
Sig: Place a 1-inch ribbon on a toothbrush; brush for 2 min daily and expectorate. Avoid rinsing or eating for 30 min following treatment.

Rx: Thera-Flur-N 1.1% gel.
Disp: 1 tube.
Sig: Place a 1-inch ribbon on a toothbrush; brush for 2 min daily and expectorate. Avoid rinsing or eating for 30 min following treatment.

Rx: Neutral NaF 1.1 % dental crm. PreviDent 5000 Plus toothpaste.
Disp: 2 oz. tube.
Sig: Place a 1-inch ribbon on a toothbrush; brush for 2 min twice daily and expectorate. Avoid rinsing or eating for 30 min following treatment.

Fluoride gels available are shown in Table 18-1.

When the taste of acidulated fluoride gels is poorly tolerated or when there is etching of ceramic restorations, neutral pH sodium fluoride gel 1% (Thera-Flur-N, PreviDent) should be considered.

FDA regulations have limited the size of bottles of fluoride owing to toxicity if ingested by infants. Since most preparations do not come in childproofed bottles, the sizes of topical fluoride preparations vary; 24 mL is approximately a 2-week supply for application to a full dentition in custom carriers.

Xerostomia, reduced salivary flow, and dry mouth provide an excellent environment for the overgrowth of *Candida albicans*. The patient is likely to require treatment for candidiosis along with the treatment for dry mouth. Refer to Chapter 2, "Candidosis."

In a dry oral environment, plaque control becomes more difficult. Meticulous oral hygiene is essential.

ADDITIONAL READINGS

Atkinson JC, Fox PC. Sjogren's syndrome: oral and dental considerations. J Am Dent Assoc 1993;124:74–86.

Cevimeline (Evoxac) for dry mouth. Med Lett Drugs Ther 2000;42:70.

Daniels TE. Sjogren's syndrome: clinical spectrum and current diagnostic controversies. Adv Dent Res 1996;10:3–8.

Ferguson MM. Pilocarpine and other cholinergic drugs in management of salivary gland dysfunction. Oral Surg Oral Med Oral Pathol 1993;75:186–91.

Fox PC. Differentiation of dry mouth etiology. Adv Dent Res 1996;10:13–6.

Greenspan D. Xerostomia: diagnosis and management. Oncology 1996;10(3 Suppl):7–11.

Grisius MM. Salivary gland dysfunction: a review of systemic therapies. Oral Surg Oral Med Oral Pathol Oral Radiol Endod 2001;92:156–62.

Navazesh M. How can oral health care providers determine if patients have dry mouth? J Am Dent Assoc 2003;134:613–20.

Navazesh M. Salivary gland hypofunction in elderly patients. J Calif Dent Assoc 1994;22:62–8.

Pajukoski H, Meurman JH, Halonen P, Sulkava R. Prevalence of subjective dry mouth and burning mouth in hospitalized elderly patients and outpatients in relation to saliva, medication, and systemic diseases. Oral Surg Oral Med Oral Pathol Oral Radiol Endod 2001;92:641–9.

Smith RG, Burtner AP. Oral side effects of the most frequently prescribed drugs. Spec Care Dent 1994;14:96–102.

Wynn RL. Oral pilocarpine (Salagen)—a recent approved salivary stimulant. Gen Dent 1996;44:26–30.

Appendix 1

SUPPORTIVE CARE

Management of oral mucosal conditions may require topical and/or systemic interventions. Therapy should address patient nutrition and hydration, oral discomfort, oral hygiene, management of secondary infection, identification of possible drug interactions, and local control of the disease process. Depending on the extent, severity, and location of oral lesions, consideration should be given to obtaining a consultation from a dentist who specializes in oral medicine, oral pathology, or oral surgery. When there is a question involving a medical condition, a physician should be consulted.

Symptomatic relief of painful conditions can be provided with topical preparations such as 2% viscous lidocaine hydrochloride or dyclonine hydrochloride throat lozenges (OTC). Topical anesthetics can be used as a rinse in adults but should be applied with a cotton swab in a child so that the child does not swallow the medication. Swallowing these anesthetics is contraindicated, in part, because they may interfere with the patient's gag reflex. Symptomatic relief can also be obtained by mixing equal parts of diphenhydramine hydrochloride elixir and magnesium hydroxide or aluminum hydroxide. Children's formula diphenhydramine hydrochloride elixir does not contain alcohol. Sucralfate suspension may also be used prior to meals. The diphenhydramine mixture and the sucralfate suspension coat the ulcerated lesions and may allow the patient to eat more comfortably.

Mouth rinses containing a hydroalcoholic vehicle should be avoided because of the oral discomfort that will result from their use. The amount of oral discomfort experienced by patients with oral mucosal lesions varies and can often be controlled without the use of narcotic analgesics. Non-narcotic analgesics are often helpful.

Meticulous oral hygiene is absolutely mandatory for these patients. Mucosal lesions contacting bacterial plaque present on the dentition are more likely to become secondarily infected. Patients should be seen by the dentist or hygienist for scaling and root planing, under local anesthesia when necessary, in all cases in which oral hygiene is suboptimal. Patients must be encouraged to brush and floss their teeth after meals in a gentle yet efficient manner. Placing a soft toothbrush under hot water to further soften the bristles may enhance this. Tartar control toothpastes containing calcium pyrophosphate should be avoided because of their irritating nature and reported involvement in circumoral dermatitis.

INDEX